The Addiction Recovery Journal

Dear Reader,

Thanks for purchasing my book.

I feel grateful to serve you with,
The Addiction Recovery Journal

And I sincerely hope you enjoy, learn
and find what you're looking for.

All the best,

CW. V. Straaten

Do you want Free Recovery Exercises?
Send an email to cw.vanstraaten@yahoo.com

Title the e-mail "366 Recovery"

And I will send you the exercises for Free.

Copyright © 2018 C.W. V. Straaten

Published by: True Potential Project

ISBN: 9781720269359

All rights reserved.

No part of this publication may be reproduced, distributed, or transmitted in any form or by any means, including photocopying, recording, or other electronic or mechanical methods, without the prior written permission of the publisher, except in the case of brief quotations embodied in critical reviews and certain other noncommercial uses permitted by copyright law. For permission requests, write to the publisher.

Disclaimer

This book is not intended to act as a substitute for medical advice or treatment. Any person with a condition requiring medical attention should consult a qualified medical practitioner or suitable therapist. The information provided in this book is stated to be truthful and consistent, in that any liability, in terms of inattention or otherwise, by any usage or abuse of any policies, processes, or directions contained within is the solitary and utter responsibility of the recipient reader. Under no circumstances will any legal responsibility or blame be held against the publisher for any reparation, damages, or monetary loss due to the information herein, either directly or indirectly.

The Addiction Recovery Journal

366 Days of Transformation, Writing & Reflection

CREATED BY:

C.W. V. STRAATEN

Instagram: become_recovery

A MESSAGE FROM THE AUTHOR.

This guided journal is created with the intention to help you during your recovery process. And to present you with guided questions and inspiration to overcome your addiction for good.

Reflection is the art of asking good questions.

Different questions.

To unravel the past.

Learn the lessons from years of suffering.

And, above all, to lay the foundation for brighter days.

INTRODUCTION

"What's the book you want to read yourself?"

A good friend and fellow author asked me this question at my birthday party. Most of the guests had already left and we were contemplating life under a clear sky. I had already written two self-help books about addiction and recovery. My reason for writing those books was to give my gambling addiction, and the recovery journey that followed, a deeper purpose. I wanted to share the lessons I learned. Now, I had numerous ideas in mind for my third book. But none of these ideas really made me enthusiastic. The next day, when I walked through a sunny park, the question posed by my friend came back to mind:

"What's the book you want to read yourself?"

After years of delving into self-development books, seminars, coaching, programs, and YouTube videos, I have realized that change begins by asking better questions. Or, at least, different questions. It leads to different answers and, almost exclusively in the long term, to better answers. Yes, questions hold enormous power. That's why one question in a certain conversation could stick with you for days. And that's why I decided in December 2017, when reflecting on the question of my friend, that creating a journal would be the best self-help book I could create. To give the reader the exact tools to go on a journey of self-discovery; a journey of reflection to learn from the past; a journey of gratitude and hopefulness; a journey to make the necessary changes, to experience the joy of daily life, and to create the life you want to live.

And thus, I created this one-year journal. Each day poses a new question or short exercise to lead you on a path of recovery, happiness, and self-improvement. With much care, I made these questions and arranged them in a specific order to create a unique journey of self-improvement. If you are recovering from an addiction, trying to quit your addiction, or wanting to examine your bad habit(s), then this journal is for you. With so much as setting aside five or ten minutes a day for using *The Addiction Recovery Journal*, you could make significant changes in your life. Not just immediate changes in how you feel, or insights about your past, but also long-term changes regarding self-acceptance and self-confidence. And, eventually, it will be your own unique recovery journal that will reveal your insights, beautiful life moments, and lessons learned. A one-year autobiography.

All in all, this is a complete Recovery Journal that guides you to brighter days.

But there is more! If you seek inspiration during the 366-days, I have created an extensive list of tips and tricks for your recovery journey that you can find at the end of this book. Also, every thirty days, there is brief advice derived from my own recovery journey.

How To Use This Journal

Every page of this book contains a new day, with a new question or short exercise. I recommend using this journal during your morning or evening routine. This way you can integrate journaling as a short, simple, and powerful daily habit.

There are similar questions, about gratitude and paying closer attention to your own qualities in this journal. I've done this to bring these topics, which we often tend to forget, into the spotlight.

In this journal, I use the word constructive/construction as the counterpart for destructive/destruction.

At the end of this journal you will find a preview of my book

The Addiction Recovery Workbook: A 7-Step Master Plan To Take Back Control Of Your Life

You can check out my other books, all intended for both personal development and recovery from addiction, here:
www.amazon.com/C-W-V-Straaten/e/B072QWFDKJ

Daily Recovery Inspirations

If you want to focus on becoming free from addiction & commit to recovery every day, follow my instagram account. With a recovery inspiration every day.

Instagram: become_recovery
https://www.instagram.com/become_recovery/.

Or you can search on C.W. V. Straaten.

Day 1

If your addiction was a person, how would you describe him or her? What is the one piece of advice you would give him or her?

Day 2

What could other people learn from you?

Day 3

What does recovery mean to you?

Day 4

What would happen if, for the next thirty days, you said no when you wanted to say no and yes when you wanted to say yes?

Day 5

30 Day Challenge. Pick a new small, constructive, and simple habit and try it for the next 30 Days. Examples: Reading for 10 minutes a day; drinking a smoothie a day; making your bed every day, or meditating for five minutes a day.

Day 6

If you would take ten percent more responsibility for your own happiness, what would happen?

Day 7

What would be a better way to deal with your hurt feelings?

Day 8

What triggers your addiction? Name up to three triggers. What are other ways to deal with these triggers

"The enemy is a very good teacher."
The Dalai Lama

Day 9

If your addiction was the enemy, what could you learn from it?

Day 10

Write down three things you can do
to deal better with setbacks in life.

> *"Insanity is doing the same thing over and over again and expecting a different result."*
> Albert Einstein

Day 11

Name three small actions you can take to calm your mind.
Do at least one of these actions today.

Day 12

Write down at least seven reasons
why your addictive behaviour is irrational.

Day 13

Write down three intelligent things you can do to prevent a relapse.

Day 14

If you had the strong belief that your decisions are under your control, how would life be different for the next seven days?

Day 15

Describe the purely evil side of your addiction. Name at least one thing / thought / person / dream that could serve as a light against the darkness of your addiction.

Day 16

Name ten things you're grateful for in life.

"At one point, we all consciously decided how much to eat and what to focus on when we got to the office, how often to have a drink or when to go for a jog. Then we stopped making a choice, and the behavior became automatic. It's a natural consequence of our neurology. And by understanding how it happens, you can rebuild those patterns in whichever way you choose."
Charles Duhigg, *The Power of Habit*

Day 17
When did your destructive habit start?

Day 18
Write down three good things you can do to deal with boredom?

Day 19

What role does procrastination play in leading up to your addictive behavior? What is one thing you could do to battle procrastination?

Day 20

What would your life look like in three months if you stay on this recovery journey? And in a year?

Day 21

What is the root cause of your addiction?

Day 22

Write down an empowering response to the addiction thought, recovery is boring.

Day 23

Has addiction been a means for you to flee from reality?
If so, what is it that scares you so much?

Day 24

What gives you hope?

Day 25

What would you want people to understand about your addiction?

Day 26

Are you afraid to let people see your true colors? Why or why not?

"The price of inaction is far greater than the cost of making a mistake."
Meister Eckhart

Day 27

What dreams have you delayed because of your addiction?

Day 28

If you allow yourself to make mistakes, what would you do differently tomorrow? And what would you have done differently in the past?

Day 29

Name 12 things you're grateful for in your life.

Day 30

What are your three best character traits?

Month 1

A Morning Ritual

During my recovery journey, I've learned many new things but none of them had such a profound impact on my life as creating a morning ritual. It is transforming to start the day by taking control of your morning. Instead of Facebook feeds or news channels claiming your attention, you control your time and prepare yourself for the day. This habit alone, which could take as long as fifteen minutes, can be a game-changer during your recovery. On Day 33 there is an exercise for creating a morning ritual. For now, here are five examples of what I do when I wake up (in chronological order):

- Write in my dream journal
- Take a shower
- Drink hot water with ginger
- Do five minutes of exercises, such as push-ups
- Write down my intention for the day: 1 or 2 major goals, and 1 or 2 minor goals

Day 31

Sometimes during an addiction binge you might have (had) the feeling of "losing it all". Somehow that doesn't always feel so frightening. In fact, it could be the thing you look forward to... Losing it all. Or, did you actually long for a new beginning?

Day 32

What does happiness mean to you?

Day 33

What would be a constructive and positive morning ritual for you?
Try it for three days.

Day 34

How often did you tell yourself, "I am worthless,"?
Is it time for another statement?

Day 35

Is there a dark side lurking beneath your surface?
If so, how do you treat it?

Day 36

Would it be an idea to meet with your dark side kindly
and let it express itself in a healthy way?

Day 37

What is the pattern that leads to your addiction?

Day 38

Write down one or two things you can do to interrupt the pattern that leads to addictive behavior.

Day 39

Write down the key lesson you learned from your addiction.

Day 40

What advice would you ten-year older self give to you now.

Day 41

Addiction has an enormous power. If that power and energy is yours, and you could use it for something constructive, it could make a huge difference in your life. For what area / specific action could you use ten percent more energy?

Day 42

If you were put on this earth for a reason, what would the reason be?

Day 43
What about last week makes you feel grateful.

Day 44
Who would you like to be one year from now?

Day 45

Describe a past experience where you overcame failure.

Day 46

What did you learn from overcoming failure in the past?

Day 47

What can you do on a daily basis that is easy, fun and positive?

Day 48

If you no longer searched for recognition, how would life be different?

"When I let go of what I am, I become what I might be."
Lao Tzu

Day 49

What did you tell yourself to become an addict?

Day 50

If you could be ten percent more positive,
how would tomorrow be different?

Day 51

Write down three things you can do to be more kind to yourself.

Day 52

Write down at least five positive experiences / insights during your recovery journey.

"Start small and keep it simple. That's our motto for change."
21 Exercises, *The Secrets For Self-Growth*

Day 53

Is a childhood wound still running your life today?
What could be the next step towards accepting and fixing it?

Day 54

What is a small step you can take right now
that will lead to a better life?

Day 55

How would your seven-year-old-self describe you?

Day 56

What is keeping you in the past?

Day 57

Are expectations holding you back
from experiencing the here and now?

Day 58

What would you like to do tomorrow?

Day 59

Write down a list with all your skills and qualities.

Day 60

How has addiction positively shaped you?

Month 2

Taking Small Steps

A lot of people who are into self-development are falling into the trap of wanting too much in a short amount of time. This willingness is where get-rich-quick gurus build a fortune on. However, lasting change doesn't happen overnight. It's an in-depth self-discovery journey combined with taking consistent small steps that lead to the big changes. It *will* take time, however. And that's okay. The journey itself is where you can focus on. And where, between hard lessons and moments of conflicts, you find joy & confidence about your silent progression.

Day 61

What advice would you give someone else in recovery?

Day 62

What is something in the past you feared but did anyway?

Day 63
What does being lonely mean to you?

Day 64
What do you look forward to in the near future?

Day 65

When was the last time you had to *pick yourself up*?
How did you do it?

Day 66

Release your worries and negative thoughts on paper.

*"God, grant me the serenity to accept the things I cannot change,
the courage to change the things I can,
and the wisdom to know the difference."*
Serenity Prayer

Day 67

What is something you have to accept?

Day 68
How did addiction trick you?

Day 69
Write down seven reasons why you believe you can recover from addiction for good..

Day 70

Write down three recent achievements that make you proud.

Day 71

What are you constantly searching for?

Day 72
What does your *Inner Voice* is trying to tell you?

Day 73
Are you validating yourself based on material things?

Day 74
What makes you a beautiful person?

Day 75
Is life trying to teach you a particular lesson? What is it?

Day 76

If a relapse happens, see it as part of the path to recovery. Write down five self-care activities you can do after a relapse.

Day 77

Are you ignoring your true calling?

Day 78

When was the last time you laughed so hard it hurt?

Day 79

Celebrate life. Treat yourself today or tomorrow with something that feels right and joyous. Write down exactly what you're going to do.

Day 80

What do you feel guilty about?
What first step could you take to forgive yourself / make it right?

Day 81

Are you still maintaining a secret life?

Day 82

How would tomorrow be different if you'd express yourself freely?

Day 83

If a writer decided to write a book about your life, what would be the genre? Comedy, drama, inspirational, etc. Why?

Day 84

When was the last time you gave someone a compliment?
Give a compliment each day, for the next week.

Day 85

Write down a list of compliments you've received in your life.

> *"To be happy we need something to solve.
> Happiness is therefore a form of action"*
> Mark Manson, *The Subtle Art of Not Giving a F*ck*

Day 86

Problems are an inevitable part of life.
What problems would you like to solve?

Day 87

What is your body trying to tell you?

Day 88

What makes you feel embarrassed?

Day 89

What is the life you deserve to live?

"Be yourself; everyone else is already taken."
Oscar Wilde

Day 90

What kind of self-talk helps you improve?

Month 3

Don't Be Too Hard On Yourself

Regret is a logical consequence of making the 'wrong' decisions in the past. Especially when these decisions became a pattern and created destruction. When you confront yourself with your past mistakes it's easy to fall into self-blame. It's good to feel these feelings. And to express them in a civilized way. But another part in this process is to take small steps towards making things better.

First of all, understand and accept that the journey of recovery is tough enough already. You don't need another enemy. You need a friend. So at the very least, be your own friend. Help yourself. And recognize the fact that deciding you want to quit your addiction and taking the small steps to do so is an enormous accomplishment. Every time someone decides to break destruction, it lights up the world.

Day 91

What would happen if you set rules about how to use your time?

Day 92

Is there a repetitive lesson adversity is trying to teach you?

"You know, sometimes all you need is twenty seconds of insane courage. Just literally twenty seconds of just embarrassing bravery. And I promise you, something great will come of it."
Benjamin Mee, We Bought A Zoo

Day 93

How would the next month be different,
if every day you had 20 seconds of insane courage?

Day 94

What actions can you take
to improve your recovery journey this week?

Day 95

What clouds your judgement?

Day 96

Write down twelve things you are grateful for in your life.

Day 97

Why did addiction arrive on your path?

Day 98

What is giving you stress?

Day 99

Why did recovery arrive on your path?

Day 100

Are there voices from other people in your head that are preventing you from living the life you want to live?

> *"Be the change that you wish to see in the world."*
> Mahatma Gandhi

Day 101
How could you better express your emotions?

Day 102
How could you train your patience?

Day 103

Meditating is one of the best ways to calm your mind and eventually better analyze your thoughts and living with more awareness.
Try to meditate this week for at least five minutes a day. Write down how and when you are going to do it.

Day 104

Write down five things you can do to deal better with stress.

Day 105

Do you feel competent enough to deal with the struggles of life?

Day 106

What void did you try to fill with your addiction?

Day 107

What values do you find important?

Day 108

What is an act of kindness you could do today / tomorrow to make someone's day? Yes... do it!

Day 109

Could you reduce the stream of negativity in your life? How can you do this on a regular basis? Try it for three days.

Day 110

What are three constructive things you could do when problems become overwhelming?

Day 111

If doing your best was good enough, how would that make you feel?

Day 112

Do you find life demanding? Why or why not?

Day 113

If you look at your life so far, what lessons did you learn?

Day 114

Is there another addiction lurking under the surface?
If so, what is it trying to fulfill?

Day 115

Describe what "living the good life" means to you.

Day 116

What patterns keep returning in when it comes to your love life?

Day 117

How would you like to be remembered?

Day 118

What patterns keep returning in your life when it comes to money?

Day 119

"If your motivation for acquiring money or success comes from a nonsupportive root such as fear, anger, or the need to "prove" yourself, your money will never bring you happiness."
T. Harv Eker, Secrets of the Millionaire Mind

Write down three actions to improve your finances this month.

Make an agreement with yourself to take at least one of these actions this month.

Day 120

"Health is the greatest possession. Contentment is the greatest treasure. Confidence is the greatest friend."
Lao Tzu

Write down three actions to improve your health this month.

Make an agreement with yourself to take at least one of these actions this month.

Month 4

Enjoy Life

It's easy to forget. Certainly amidst every day's troubles, certainly amidst the struggles of recovery. But it's important to hold still for a while. To realize the gift of life. To breathe it in. To look around. To feel it. That spirit of life, of flow, of love. This doesn't mean to be positive all the time. It means to pay attention. To things, people, experiences. We tend to take them for granted so easily. Paying attention and being grateful could turn all these ordinary and dull moments into something a bit more extraordinary.

Day 121

In what direction is your life heading?

Day 122

What fear / doubt is constantly blocking you from taking the necessary actions? Is it worth it?

Day 123
What is distracting you?

Day 124
Write down three things that could improve your overall energy.

Day 125

What are five goals you absolutely want to achieve this year. If you had to choose only one of these goals, which would it be?

Day 126

Do something joyous / exciting within two weeks that feels right. It doesn't have to be expensive and could be as small as treating yourself to a Netflix night. Write it down, schedule it in your agenda and make sure to follow through.

Day 127

How could you connect with your Higher Self on a regular basis?

Day 128

Write down three things you can do to improve your self-confidence.

Day 129

What has journaling brought you so far?

Day 130

What is making you sad? And, what is making you happy?

Day 131

Is there a more intelligent way to deal with your impulses?

Day 132

What would happen if you did the opposite for the next 24 hours?

Day 133
How can you still accomplish your greatest dream(s)?

Day 134
What motivates you to get out of bed in the morning?

Day 135

Are you too hard on yourself?

Day 136

Is it difficult for you to make decisions?
If so, what makes it so difficult?

*"If you look the right way,
you can see that the whole world is a garden."*
Frances Hodgson Burnett

Day 137

In what area of your life do you need to pay more attention?

Day 138

Write down how other people, books, programs, can help you with these solutions.

Day 139

What has your childhood taught you?

Day 140

Did your addiction serve a purpose?

Day 141

What is standing between your dreams and reality?

Day 142

How could you listen better to your own needs?
What would happen if you did?

Day 143

What would happen if you were more kind to the people around you?

Day 144

Are you still afraid of your addiction?
If so, what could you do to be less afraid?

> *"I can't give you a sure-fire formula for success, but I can give you a formula for failure: try to please everybody all the time."*
> Herbert Bayard Swope

Day 145

Is life going by too fast? What could you do to pay more attention?

Day 146

Is there something you still need to do?

Day 147

What lesson did you learn about yourself in the past few months?

Day 148

Is money ruling your life, or do you rule money?

Day 149

If you had one hour more each day, what would you do with it? Could you create an extra hour a day?

Day 150

How would you describe integrity?

Month 5

You're Not Always Right

During the road of recovery, you discover lots of new insights. Sometimes this is frightening, because it means you have to reevaluate your old beliefs. It could mean that you were not right. And actually, to me, that was one of the most fascinating parts of my recovery journey. The discovery of a new thought, a new belief. It helped me to grow. Grow away from my past. Put a healthy distance between me and these low vibration thoughts and sensations. Traveling new roads leads to new discoveries. Be open to it. If you want or have to change your life, new beliefs are mandatory.

Day 151

Do you lack integrity in your life?
If so, where? And what is the reason for it?

Day 152

Does your impatience have something to do
with how much you trust your own capacities?

Day 153

Success is most of the time as scary or even scarier than staying where you are. We all want a million dollars... But do we?

Isn't this kind of success, or to achieve the goals you set for yourself, not an unconscious bridge too far?

Are the goals you set for yourself what you really want?

Try to discuss with yourself the doubts you have about your goals.

Is it worth letting these doubts dictate your life?

Day 154

What could you do to prepare yourself for better times / success?

Day 155

Are the unconscious doubts you have about reaching your goals coming from low self-esteem? (Do I really deserve to be loved / make more money / do what I am passionate about / be happy?)

Day 156
Are you on the right track?

Day 157
Name three ways to feel more attractive. What is one action you can do today / tomorrow to feel more attractive?

Day 158

When did you feel abandoned?

Day 159

What can you say to that version of you who felt abandoned?

Day 160

How can you make a difference
in the lives of those around you this week?

Day 161

To whom do you often compare yourself to? Why?

Day 162

What are you afraid of / worried about in the near future? Analyze this fear / worry. Could you accept it? If not, what could you do to prepare yourself for the worst outcome?

Day 163

What is it about yourself that you hope other people won't find out?

Day 164

How could you allow success to happen?

Day 165

Are you growing and evolving, or are you actually staying under the same ceiling? If so, why is that?

Day 166

Do you need to accept or to change?

Day 167

How can you take (better) care of your most precious talent(s)?

Day 168

Could it be that it is scarier for you to be accepted than to be rejected?

Day 169

What would you like to learn in the next three months?

Day 170

When was the last time you surprised yourself?

Day 171

Could you accept a compliment?

Day 172

Is it difficult for you to tell the truth? If so, what makes it difficult?

Day 173

What things in life do you take for granted?

Day 174

Describe the first moment you realized you want to recover from addiction for good.

Day 175

Do you feel you deserve to be a recovered addict? Why or why not?

*"How can you waste time? You have only so much to use,
and no matter what you do, it still passes."*
Felix Salten

Day 176
What emotions are paralyzing you?

Day 177
Is your ambition coming from your soul / heart or your ego?

Day 178

Are you eager to live a better life?

Day 179

Write down three reasons or more why you fundamentally disagree with everything addiction stands for.

"It takes courage to grow up and become who you really are."
E.E. Cummings

Day 180

Do you need a vacation?
If so, why?

Month 6

Relaxation

Working on yourself can be overwhelming. Taking action on your goals, working on your health, finances, social life, all of that: it demands your time and energy. But that's not it. You have your work and other every day obligations. A vital part is finding harmony in once life. Relaxation is one of the keys to balance out work and effort. Try to take a moment for yourself every day, or share a moment with your loved ones, where you just *be*. Enjoy these moments, hours, days. Why not give relaxation as much importance as effort. Try to find how harmony works for you.. Resting isn't without value; it's the time you take, to refresh.

Day 181

How would someone else describe you during an addiction episode?

Day 182

What could you do this week to improve your financial situation? Make the commitment to yourself to follow through on this action.

Day 183

Where in your actions / thoughts are you contradicting yourself?

Day 184

Again, write down an empowering morning routine that would help you to start your day great. Try this new morning routine for seven days.

Day 185

What one thing can you do today to reach your most important goal?

Day 186

Do you miss love in your life? If so, make the commitment to yourself to give love to others for the next seven days.

Day 187

Write down the negative feelings / emotions that you would do almost anything to avoid?

Day 188

What life lessons would you give to a class of sixteen year olds?

Day 189

Where in your life do you need guidance?
How can you find this guidance?

Day 190

How do you see your addiction now? What is the main lesson you learned about your addiction in the past month?

Day 191

Is your social circle improving your life?

Day 192

If you could be with your twelve year old self for one day, what would you do? And what would you say?

"Most folks are about as happy as they make up their minds to be."
Abraham Lincoln

Day 193

See today's quote. Is this true for you? Why or why not?

Day 194

Is your Inner Child still alive? How do you recognize him or her?

Day 195

Name one little achievement that has had a big impact on your life.

Day 196

If you could clean up your mind, where would you begin

Day 197

Look in the mirror right now, and ask yourself the question: *"Is what I am doing every day fulfilling?"* What would your answer be?

Day 198

What makes you feel self-confident?

Day 199

How did your life look like exactly one year ago? Write down the progress you've made so far, and... be grateful for it.

Day 200

What does being a significant, successful person mean to you?

Day 201

What skill(s) do you need to improve, to live the life you want to live?

Day 202

If you could be with your four year old self for one day, what would you do?

Day 203

Is there something you *need* from other people?
Could you try to *give* it yourself first?

Day 204

In the last three months, what (small) changes
have you seen in your life?

Day 205

Why are you still on this recovery journey?

Day 206

What is your plan for the next month?

Day 207

What is the one thing you could do today/tomorrow to improve your relationship with your family / best friends?

Day 208

What is the one thing you could do today/tomorrow to improve the relationship with yourself?

Day 209

Write down an empowering response to the addiction thought, Addiction has ruined my future.

Day 210

What is your biggest *"Why"* for the things you do?

Month 7

Stay Inspired

Your life is in constant motion. Goals and new habits, could quickly fade away due to every day tensions. When you're unaware for a prolonged period of time, you can get sucked into a life you don't want. One way to dodge this bullet is to stay inspired. This can be done through daily journaling, proper relaxation, and giving your mind a healthy diet of inspirational content, conversations and thoughts. Because inspiration, most of the time, isn't given to you; you have to seek it. And even if it is just there: you have to allow it to land.

Day 211

What did you learn about recovery this week?

Day 212

Write down three things you can do
to practice authentic self-expression?

Day 213
What one small victory did you accomplish today?

Day 214
Write down five self-care actions you can do on a regular basis.

Day 215

What would happen if from now on, you put yourself first?

Day 216

What statements can you make about your addiction after all the time it has been in your life?

"To go fast, go alone. To go far, go together."
African proverb

Day 217

How could you better connect with other people?

Day 218

How could you inspire others?

Day 219

What voices in your head are you ignoring? Could it be that this / these voice(s) have an important message to tell you?

Day 220

What could you do today/tomorrow
to improve your most important skills?

Day 221

New habit challenge. Is it possible for you to integrate a new, small habit in your life for 30 days? Pick something that could be a game changer, but won't cost a lot of effort, and write it down. Examples: Making your bed, daily goal setting in the morning (one major and one minor goal), an apple a day, 10 / 15 sit ups each day.

Day 222

What is something new you could try this week?

Day 223

What is still lurking under the surface, that needs to be addressed?

Day 224

Are you still blaming certain people for past experiences? What small steps can you take in the coming months to forgive them?

Day 225

What are you blessed with in your life?

Day 226

What has your addiction taught you about yourself?

Day 227

Is there something you should say yes to in the next month?

Day 228

Write down an empowering response to the addiction thought, *I am never able to fully control my addiction.*

Day 229

Describe your comfort zone when it comes to finances?

Day 230

Describe your comfort zone
when it comes to your love life/dating life?

Day 231

Write down a list of material things you actually no longer need.

Day 232

In what ways are you a different person now than the person who was heavily addicted?

Day 233

Write down a list of small actions you can take that will have a significant effect on your long term well-being.

Day 234

Is there a version of yourself trying to claw its way out?

Day 235

If you would receive $1000 today, how would you spend it?

Day 236

What would happen
if you were ten percent more proactive in your life?

Day 237

Is your addictive craving genuinely fading? Why or why not?

Day 238

What is triggering you towards inauthentic behavior or thoughts?

Day 239

What problems in your life are actually opportunities?

Day 240

How would your ideal day for tomorrow look like?
What's stopping you?

Month 8

Exciting Goals

In times of boredom, procrastination or when you're about to give up, the purpose behind your goals (*the why*) can help you to get through. One of my goals was to live for three months in South America. The thoughts, images surrounding that dream, made it quite easy for me to do the work that would allow me to make that jump. It's about excitement. That fuels your work ethos. It colors your life. What are you excited about? What is your motivation to get out of bed? Make it a part of your goals. Create an exciting future for yourself that you would like to walk into every day.

Day 241

Are you living a life true to your potential?

Day 242

What do people see when you walk into a room?

Day 243

What lies did you tell yourself in order to keep going with your addictive behavior?

Day 244

What would happen this week if you were ten percent more assertive?

Day 245

How would you describe the feeling of powerlessness you've felt towards addiction? Write down also at least one reason why this powerlessness is simply not true.

Day 246

What troubles do you have in your life right now that will seem meaningless ten years from now?

Day 247

How would your most courageous, self-confident, kindest and strongest self look like? What advice would he/she give to you?

Day 248

Which area in your life needs attention? Take at least 15 minutes a day for the next three days to give the proper attention to this area.

Day 249

What can other people learn from you when it comes to recovery from addiction?

Day 250

What do you find stupid now about addiction?

Day 251

Write down five reasons why you know addiction will never have that power over your life again.

Day 252

What do you associate with an authentic life, one without secrets?

Day 253

Are you taking yourself too seriously sometimes? Why and when?

Day 254

How is your true self, different from the version of you during your periods of addiction?

Day 255

How can humility help you in accepting yourself?

Day 256

Write down a list of all the people in your life that you feel grateful for.

Day 257

How can you connect with the Universe / Infinite Wisdom, or God?

Day 258

How could you be a guide for yourself?

Day 259

What would you like to learn about dealing with conflict?

*"It's no use going back to yesterday,
because I was a different person then."*
Lewis Carroll

Day 260

When did you feel ignored?
What can you say to that version of you who felt ignored?

Day 261

Write down two or three recent memories when you felt truly peaceful.

Day 262

One or two times strangers helped you in unexpected ways.

Day 263

How could you work smarter instead of harder?

Day 264

Who is inspiring you? Why?

Day 265

How could you cultivate kindness in your life?

Day 266

Are you surrounding yourself with the right people?
Is there someone missing?

Day 267

If you would meet your sixteen year old self today, what would he / she look like? What would you tell him or her about the future? And what advice would you give?

Day 268

Who are you judging too much?

Day 269

What social conditions are suppressing you?

Day 270

You are not your addiction, nor your recovery. What is your true purpose here on earth?

Month 9

Meditation

Your thoughts hold an enormous power on your overall well-being. Left unexamined, they decide your destiny in life. When you can control your mind, anything is possible. Controlling thoughts, however, requires work. Sit still for one minute and pay attention to your rushing thoughts. They go anywhere, demanding you to go with them. Even if they go to places of anger, frustration, craving, worry or sadness.

The best way to regain control over your thoughts is through meditation. Meditation is the art of paying attention, increasing your awareness, and letting go. On Day 104 you were given a short meditation exercise. Hopefully, you've already made it part of your daily or weekly routine. It can make a significant difference in your long time happiness and success, but it will also give you an immediate feeling of calmness and joy. A double reward.

Day 271

How is your image different from your authentic self?

Day 272

Why is it scary to drop the *image*?

Day 273

What would happen if you'd be ten percent more vulnerable in the conversations with your best friends and/or family?

Day 274

What can you do this week to improve your overall health?

Day 275

Write down a memory, where you did everything to be in total control, but then it seemed you weren't in control after all.

Day 276

What would happen in a year, if:
You would hold yourself to a ten percent higher standard?
You would hold yourself to a ten percent lower standard?

> *"I don't know half of you half as well as I should like; and I like less than half of you half as well as you deserve."*
> J.R.R. Tolkien, The Fellowship of the Ring

Day 277

What does it take to gain your trust?

Day 278

Do you trust yourself? Why or why not?

Day 279

What about addiction did you love? What other activities can give you these same benefits in a healthy way?

Day 280

Which doubts require your attention?

Day 281

Name three experiences in your life where you let fear dictate your decisions and became disappointed with the result.

Day 282

What have others liked about you, that you didn't notice yourself?

Day 283

How could you bring more joy into your life?

Day 284

Be so kind and generous to spend $5–$50 this week to treat yourself. Write down what you're going to do and when you're going to do it.

Day 285

Are your goals motivating you or are they giving you stress?

Day 286

What inner conflict needs your attention?

"When in doubt, just take the next small step."
Paulo Coelho

Day 287

What is your next small step?

Day 288

When was the last time you expressed yourself authentically? How did it feel?

Day 289

What self-image did your childhood give you?

Day 290

A list of things that make you smile.

Day 291

What action would the next best version of you take when it comes to your career/business?

Day 292

What new places in or around your hometown can you visit this year?

Day 293
What one small victory did you accomplish this week?

Day 294
Are there thoughts that are still blocking the quality of your life? How can you deal with these thoughts?

Day 295

What are one or three favorite memories from your childhood?

Day 296

Is something in your recovery irritating you?
If so, what small steps can you take today to solve it?

Day 297

Reflect on the relationship you have with yourself.
What is good about it? What can you do better?

Day 298

Write down three things you can do to improve your charisma?

Day 299

What are you excited about in your life right now?

Day 300

What does it say about addiction, that you need so many secrets in order to keep continuing doing it?

Month 10

The Magic Sparkle Of Connection

We tend to be most grateful for the moments we share with other people. Friends, family, acquaintances, colleagues, even strangers. When you truly connect with someone else, there is this sparkle of magic. It does good to take care of these connections. By paying attention when you are interacting. To see the other as a whole human being. To be present. To listen. And to speak authentically. Also, try to take care about your existing relationships. Don't take them for granted. Take care of them, as you would take care of a lovely garden. Is it time to have that much needed heart-to-heart talk with your loved one? Or do you still need to thank a good friend? Reunite with an old acquaintance?

When I look back on my addiction years, one of the saddest memories is the overall loneliness I felt. The secrets, the lies, the shame that led to these moments of solitary existence. Of isolation. During my recovery journey, I made it my first commitment to heal the bond with myself. To find a way to finally accept myself. Because of my financial situation, I wasn't able to go out much during my recovery. During the many nights sitting alone in my apartment and working on myself, I always felt a whispering sense of loneliness. Although I knew I was on the right track, the one thing missing was connection. Looking out the window and seeing a young couple kissing, holding hands... I felt like an outsider. Not just to the young couple, but to the rest of the world. I was constantly listening to *Fast Car*, hearing Tracy Chapman singing,

> *And your arm felt nice wrapped 'round my shoulder*
> *I had a feeling that I belonged*

I didn't belong. Or, so I thought. But then it dawned on me, why should people come to me? And actually, they did come to me. Asking me to go out. To join them. But I was too afraid to admit that I didn't have the money to go out. I was digging my own grave.

That night I decided to not just make the commitment to create a better bond with myself, but to create a better bond with others as well. To give what I sought. And to accept, receive when it was shared with me. I firmly believe that life is not meant to live alone. I believe that you project to others the relationship you have with yourself. So my lack of self-acceptance at that time made me feel uncomfortable to be with people. With or without having the money to join them. It was like a mirror. When I started to reach out, I realized once again how lucky I was with my friends and family. And how warm and intriguing it is to meet new people and feel this magic sparkle of connection.

Day 301

What small things can you do to make your living space more enjoyable?

Day 302

Does it bother you to talk about your addiction? Why, or why not?

Day 303

What childhood achievements still makes you proud today?
Try to recall one or two achievements.

Day 304

If you died today, what would you regret not doing?

Day 305

What could you give of yourself to improve the world?

Day 306

What is one decision you are still putting off?

Day 307

Write down seven reasons why you are a special person.

Day 308

Where in your life do you still recognize patterns of your addiction?

Day 309

Name three of the best experiences you've had last month.

Day 310

Would you rather be in someone's else's shoes? Why or why not?

Day 311

What is life trying to tell you at this very moment?

Day 312

If everything in life has a reason, and everything that happened to bring you where you are right now, then what is your next move?

Day 313

What recent experience caught you off guard?

Day 314

What is your favorite way to deal with social anxiety? What could be a better way to deal with it?

Day 315

If you're still doing your daily journaling: that's quite an accomplishment. If you'd like, send me a short email about your experience with this journal and how your recovery journey is going so far. My email is: cw.vanstraaten@yahoo.com. For today, write down a short recap of your journaling experience so far.

Day 316

What promises would you like to hold?

Day 317

Is lying / having secrets (still) a big part of your life?

Day 318

If you died today, what would you regret not saying?

Day 319

What advice would you give to someone who is about to relapse?

> *"Nobody has ever measured,
> not even poets, how much the heart can hold."*
> Zelda Fitzgerald

Day 320

What could be your blind spots?

Day 321

Could you challenge yourself more?
Or, should you be more appreciative of stability?

Day 322

If you could eliminate one thing from your life today, what would it be? Why?

Day 323

What simple pleasures did you enjoy this week?

Day 324

What are your mind's favorite ways to stop, belittle or diminish your enthusiasm?

Day 325

Is it difficult for you to tell someone you love him or her? Do you dare to take the following challenge: Tell someone, with all honesty, that you love him or her within the next seven days.

Day 326

What is your greatest struggle in life?
How could you help yourself to deal with this struggle?

Day 327

What would you want someone to say to you now?

Day 328
Why is vulnerability significant for self-improvement?

Day 329
What makes you proud of yourself when you reflect on last week?

Day 330

How would the best version of yourself approach your financial situation?

Day 331

How would the best version of yourself approach your social life?

Month 11

Take Care Of Your Finances

Throughout this book there are exercises to improve your financial situation. Money is a vulnerable topic to talk about. For a lot of people, money has some sort of association with evilness. I personally believe that the lack of money is the root of all evil. From top to bottom it's greed for money that does no good. The good lies in between.

Money is neutral. You can do great things with money, like building a hospital. You can do destructive things with money: like bombing the hospital. It is an energy mover. Establishing a healthy relationship with money is what you should seek. An income that suits your monthly expenses, a steady and ever-growing savings account and/or investment account & an accurate monthly plan to pay off your debts. Paying attention to your finances and making it grow (reaping and sowing) is a fine and stable foundation for living the life you want to live. Don't let the lack of money ruin your life. And start aligning to the abundance that's already all around you.

Day 332

If you treated the actions you fear as experiments, what would happen?

Day 333

What action could you take this week to improve your self-confidence? Put it in your calendar and follow through.

Day 334

What or who do you need to stay on your chosen path?

Day 335

What role does ego play in your life?

"At the bottom of her heart, however, she was waiting for something to happen. ... But each morning, as she awoke, she hoped it would come that day; she listened to every sound, sprang up with a start, wondered that it did not come; then at sunset, always more saddened, she longed for the morrow."
Gustave Flaubert, *Madame Bovary*

Day 336

What fantasies make you feel melancholic?

Day 337

Is there an area / decision in your life where your ego prevents you from living the life you want to live?

Day 338

Is it time to say goodbye to some of your dreams?
If so, which ones?

Day 339

What is your role in making the world a better place?

Day 340

In what area(s) of your life do you blindly follow the majority?

Day 341

What qualities do you despise in other people?

Day 342

What patterns are showing up repeatedly
when it comes to your social life?

Day 343

What is making your recovery journey unique and inspirational?

Day 344

If courageously dealing with an addiction is a superpower, what else could you do with this *superpower*?

> *"Reasons come first, answers come second."*
> Anthony Robbins

Day 345

What is the reason behind your three most important goals?

Day 346

What answer have you been waiting on for years?

Day 347

Are you still identifying yourself as an addict? Why or why not?

Day 348

When was the last time you tried to change something and succeeded? What is the lesson of this experience?

Day 349

If you felt safe enough to be who you really are,
how would tomorrow be different?

Day 350

What sadness held within do you need to support?

Day 351

The way you do one thing is the way you do everything.
What lessons can you learn from your current financial situation?

Day 352

Who are you?

Day 353

In what areas of your life are you walking your talk?

Day 354

The way you do one thing is the way you do everything. What lessons can you learn from your current love or dating life?

*"Forget all the reasons it won't work
and believe the one reason that it will."*
Unknown

Day 355
What pulls you through?

Day 356
What could you do when you lack motivation?

Day 357

Write down ten things you are grateful for in your life right now.

Day 358

How could you spend your time more wisely?

Day 359

What is the one message you would share with the rest of the world?

_____
_____
_____
_____
_____
_____
_____
_____
_____
_____
_____

Day 360

Write down a list of three things that you actually need, but don't own.

_____
_____
_____
_____
_____
_____
_____
_____
_____
_____
_____

Month 12

It Has Been

Through sadness and tears,
there shines a small and ever glowing light.
The dark days have been and will be,
but never it is dark enough to dim the light.
It's in you.
It's above you.
It's around you.

A faraway cry, echoing in the dark,
A child, a teenager, a you lost in time, alone, someplace, somewhere.
But time, being a strange thing, goes back and forth.
Now you, strong, brave and full of life
gives your hand to her, to him,
lonesome waiting in the past

A kind word, an arm wrapped around your shoulder
brings you back to the present

It has been, it has been.

Day 361

If you would meet a lonesome stranger, on a lonesome night, what is the one thing you would tell him about yourself?

Day 362

What has made it all worth it?

Day 363

Look in the mirror right now,
what is the one compliment you want to give yourself?

Day 364

If you met your addiction today for a last time,
what would you say to it?

Day 365

How could you be your own best friend for the coming year?

Day 366

What one question still needs to be addressed?

Preview of:

The Addiction Recovery Workbook:
A 7-Step Master Plan To Take Back Control Of Your Life

If you're interested in buying the book you can find it on Amazon.com,

A Message From The Author

"I've written this workbook first and foremost for you, the struggling addict. I wrote it because I know from experience that it can destroy your life. I wrote it because I can't stand to see so many wonderful souls being torn down by the devilish claws of addiction. I wrote it because I know there can be a way out. Even for the worst struggling addict."

"A man who can't bear to share his habits is a man who needs to quit them."

Stephen King, *The Dark Tower*

The Claws of Addiction

That you may live every day of your life.
Jonathan Swift

On the surface there was nothing wrong with me. I was renting my own apartment, had a decent job, and a kind face for almost everyone. Each day I went to work, where I behaved like a decent employee. Every weekend I went out with friends and, on more than one occasion, had a few too many drinks. But everyone does, right? I was nice to my family, nice to my neighbours, nice to unknown people in the street. But when I returned to my apartment and locked the door and closed the curtains, I was confronted with my secrets. The debts that kept piling up, loneliness, boredom, and the one solution that numbed all of my problems.

During the Christmas holidays, I had a week off. It was supposed to be a fun time. Days where you don't have to do anything. Socializing with friends, seeing your grandparents for a change, cleaning your room and reading that one book that you've looked forward to for months. All the while the atmosphere in the streets is one of kindness and warmth. Christmas is coming and everyone seems a bit more friendly. Peaceful, but I couldn't see it since the curtains of my apartment were closed.

I was constantly checking my bank account, waiting for the extra salary I was getting in December. It was the 24th of December and I was laying in my bed in my messy apartment with three empty beer cans on my desk, with a pair of trousers and my new, expensive shirt on the ground. I was looking at my phone. 3:11 PM. The money would be there at any moment. And I needed it. Oh, I desperately needed it. No more than one hour ago did I lose over 300 Euros betting on Dutch soccer. I didn't have a single dime left, not even to buy some Christmas presents. When my salary came in, all of these problems would be solved and I could finally sing along to Paul McCartney's *Wonderful Christmastime*.

One hour later. Most stores were almost closed. I had to hurry, but I was watching a live soccer match. One more goal and I would win almost 500 Euros. I was still in my bed. The curtains were still closed. It could have been the first of February, or the 13th of October. Does time matter in the hour of desperation? In the distance I heard an ambulance and the notes of a well known Christmas melody. I needed one goal. It would solve my financial situation. It would solve my depression. It would solve everything.

Three minutes were left to play. I thought about my family, I thought about the calmness, the serene feelings that were coming along with these days. And boy, did I want to be a part of it. Time was ticking indifferently. It's unbelievable to believe that you could lose an entire paycheck within one hour. You could lose everything you hold dear, for that matter, within one hour. Addiction has the enormous power to destroy conscientiousness and sensibility. It is a storm that could destroy what one has built up for months within mere minutes.

A shout, a curse. A slap against the wall. It's time. No goal. No money. No solution anymore. I watch my laptop screen in agony. The screen turns black: the live stream is over. I check my account balance, just to be certain. There it is, an indifferent, cold zero.

Your Lowest Point In Life

We addicts, or people with seriously detrimental bad habits, all know of situations like this. Maybe not as dramatic, or maybe way more dramatic. We know the stories of the husband that steals his children's college money to feed his gambling habits, or a mother that continues to drug herself while raising her children, or the boss who sexually intimidates his employees. Tough stories that speak to the imagination. It's what we link addiction to. Alcohol, drugs, gambling, sex.

But what about the millions of people who suffer from bad habits in the confidence and security of their own homes?

Housewives playing Facebook games for hours a day, the young professional who binge watches Netflix every night, the young student who spends entire days checking social media. And so on. These habits might seem a bit more trivial, but they all have the same effect: you don't see the real problem any more.

Every bad habit and every addiction serves a purpose. It grants you instantaneous pleasure. You can attain it without much effort. It won't take any effort to grab a fourth beer on Tuesday night, eat your third piece of apple pie in the middle of the night, or play that video game. (Only in the last stages of a destroying addiction does it become difficult to continue the habit, due to either a lack of money, the possibility that others might find out, or because you've made it difficult for yourself to continue. For example, not being in control of your own money anymore).

> **"People are not meant to be on this earth**
> **just to fight an addiction."**

Back to my gambling story. Unfortunately that wasn't the last time I gambled, but it was one of my last episodes. I've lost tens of thousands of Euros over my seven years of gambling. I lost an insane number of hours aimlessly watching live sporting streams in the middle of night, tired and irritated while losing over and over again. There were points where continuing to smile seemed to be an option no more. Times where I couldn't see the near future.. But somehow, whenever I woke up the next day I always had a feeling that this couldn't be what life was all about. That this wasn't the purpose. That there should be more. Much, much more. No, people are not meant to be on this earth just to fight an addiction.

It was only when I truly understood why I gambled, and when I could replace my addictive thoughts and behaviour with positive and constructive ones that disrupted the addictive pattern that real and lasting changes occurred. Now, I haven't gambled in over four years. My life has gone from debt, loneliness, and a messy apartment with closed curtains, to a rich and fulfilled life. I've used the strategy that I used to break my addiction to break other bad habits (which means either stopping it altogether or simply refraining from overindulging), such as drinking too much on a Saturday night and watching over two hours a day of television.

Now I want to share the strategy that worked successfully for me, with the rest of the world.

I've written this workbook, first and foremost, for you, the struggling addict. I wrote it because I know from experience that it can destroy your life. I wrote it because I can't stand to see so many wonderful souls being torn down by the devilish claws of addiction. I wrote it, because I know there is a way out. Even for the worst struggling addict.

Just quitting your addiction is one thing. It is what you get back when you quit or no longer overindulge in something that you feel true joy. Besides the incredible change in my financial situation, health, productivity, and social life, the change I am most excited about is the change in my consciousness. Finally, I feel strong, secure and self-confident enough to experience life fully. I'm no longer in my head all the time, which allows me to finally connect with the people I love so much, as well as new people. I can enjoy the fruits of life with integrity, as I can respond to any personal problems in a strong and constructive manner. This feeling of control, of enjoying life and most importantly, of truly connecting with other people, is worth every struggle that the gambling addiction brought to my life.

This workbook is not only intended to help you with quitting your addiction. It is also intended to help you to start over. To create and *live* the life you deserve.

Because, after all, don't you at least deserve to experience a bit more joy than the chains of addiction?

How to Read This Workbook

With this step-by-step workbook, I want to inspire and help you to take back control over your own life by not letting addiction be the guiding force of your life anymore. This book shares the same 7 simple steps I went through to quit my destructive habit: gambling addiction. I made it a structured and practical workbook that is intended to help you instantly or at the very least inspire you to take the steps necessary for you. The book guides you into the better understanding of your addiction. The reason why addiction is present in your life. Most importantly, this workbook will give you tools to solve problems your addiction has caused and to be proactive in creating a meaningful, joyful life. A life where you will be strong and secure enough to deal with the inevitable problems of life. And where you will deal with these problems consciously, without hiding in the horrific claws of addiction.

The time indicated under the steps is, of course, a mere indication. It could help to follow this timetable, in order to make your addiction process more attainable. If for whatever reason you won't go cold turkey or your goal is only to stop overindulging in your addictive behaviour, I absolutely welcome you aboard. I want to inspire you to take back control of your life. For almost all addicts that eventually means quitting altogether. But it's up to you. Take your time if you need it.

As we all know, recovery doesn't simply require the fulfillment of some steps.

Especially when accounting for the processes of revealing what kind of feelings you are trying to hide by turning to your addiction, recovery is a procedure that could take months. And for some much, much longer. But even in a shorter period of time, you can take giant steps to proactively deal with the consequences of your addiction, building up inner strength to combat your addictive cravings. And most importantly you can find meaning in your life by working on your talents, connecting with others and enjoying life to the fullest.

Note to the Reader

As stated in the disclaimer, this book is not intended to act as a substitute for medical advice or treatment. Any person with a condition requiring medical attention should consult a qualified medical practitioner or suitable therapist. Addiction can sometimes become physical, especially when you have a severe alcohol or drug addiction. Also when suffering from severe mental problems, it is wise to contact a suitable therapist. Listen to yourself and to your body, and never be too proud to ask for help.

A book is merely a book. Words are merely words. In and of themselves, they bear no magic. But you, within yourself, have the power to transform words. Into hope. Into better thoughts. Into better actions. And eventually, into change.

Don't be discouraged when you don't see overnight results. Because that's not the purpose of this book. And, I guess, that's not the purpose of any recovery method. Addiction is a giant that can only be taken down by small steps. If the only thing you get out of this book is a clearer and stronger intent on why you want to quit your addiction and how you're going to do it, that's perfectly fine.

For some this book, these words will bring more. Discover what it brings to you. And remember, don't be too hard for yourself. Please don't. A little love to yourself can go a long way. It is the announcement of a new dawn. And I sincerely hope that this book will help you to find that new dawn. To eventually stop addiction. Put an end to it. Find recovery. And then, find a new life. Your life.

Step 1. Quitting The Pattern

Day 1

***

The first step in your journey to a new life without addiction is a simple one. Just don't do it anymore. Don't smoke your cigarette anymore, stop going to the casino, stop overeating. Simple, right?

Simple, yes. Easy, no. Not at all.

Quitting your addiction might as well be one of the hardest things in the world. It means conquering an ingrained habit. It means changing something that you've been doing day in and day out, for a long period of time. It has become second nature. And whatever we say about addiction, it is something that has helped you enormously over the last few years. It has protected you when you needed it most. The addiction numbed your deep feelings of pain. But since you've purchased this workbook, you and I both know that those days are numbered. No longer is the addiction the solution. The addiction is an even worse place, despite its distraction from your deepest pains. Today will be the first step on your journey to change. Wake up from this nightmare. Meet your new dan.

In step 1 of this workbook we will go over these 4 points that will help quit your addictive pattern. These can very well be the start of your new, addiction-free life.

Quitting our addiction? Do it smart.
- **Share your story.**
- **Stop.**
- **Seek help.**
- **Cut off resources.**

Quitting your addiction? Do it smart.

This is really important. As stated in the disclaimer and in the note to the reader, this book is not intended to act as a substitute for medical advice or treatment. Take this statement to heart. Going cold turkey isn't always safe when your addiction has become physical, such as in cases of alcohol or drugs. Keep this in mind. I was a heavy gambler, a true addict. I've tried to lessen my gambling behaviour before, but at a certain moment that simply wasn't helpful anymore. The only solution for me was to quit altogether. Find your way. Be honest with yourself. Quitting your addiction? Do it smart. And it's you who, deep inside, always knows best.

Share, stop and seek help.

One of the biggest breakthroughs I had during my recovery process was sharing my story. It was just after I had made an attempt to quit gambling altogether. This unfortunately wasn't my last attempt, but the sharing of my story was crucial in eventually conquering my addiction for good. It was on a Wednesday night, just the day before I went through a long and devastating gambling period. I lost almost 2000 Euros, which was a lot of money for me at that time. When I woke up the following day, I decided – no more! That night I called one of my dear friends. After some preliminary chit chat, I was finally courageous enough to share the real reason for my phone call.

"I have a problem, and it's been going on for quite some time now. It's a gambling problem."

I was at my parents' house at the time. Nobody was home. I remember walking through the house while telling the story. My friend listened, as the very best of friends tend to do, and he offered help. It was after one more relapse that I decided to take his help. Yet sharing my addiction story was one of the best feelings I had during those dark years of gambling. It lifted the weight off my back and eventually reassured me that I didn't have to be on this journey all by myself.

That's why my advice is to share your story.

It will take courage, but it will be a huge step to freedom – to breaking down your addiction. If there is someone in your life that you can share it with, someone that won't judge you, then that just might be the person to which you can tell your story. But practice the conversation in your head. This will make it easier when you have to do it in real life. Additionally, discussing the issue over a phone call might be easier than doing it face to face. If you don't have a friend, family member or someone else to call, share it somewhere else. There are online forums or Facebook groups for people with your addiction, where you can share your story either anonymously or not. Alternatively, you could share it with a professional, anonymously with a professional helpline (telephone or chat), or a support group.

This first step, like any other first step, could easily be the most difficult one. Sharing your dark, long-kept secret may be one of the most challenging hurdles you'll ever overcome. And it's worth the struggle. By sharing it, the heavy pressure of your addiction will feel lighter, and all of a sudden you're not alone in your fight anymore.

Stop.

If you want to quit your addiction, there is no other way than to first say: 'It's over now, I'll quit.' Even if your purpose is only to lessen your addictive behaviour (for example by only gambling once per week with a specific budget, smoking three cigarettes a day, or drinking only two glasses of alcohol and only on the weekend), it's a great first step to stop altogether with your addictive behaviour for a period of time. It's crucial to be one hundred percent behind your decision to quit. If you're a spiritual person, it will help to ask your God for help in this process. If you're not spiritual, ask your Higher Self to guide and guard you in the quitting process.

The conscious decision of quitting your addiction, and actually stopping your addictive behaviour, are steps that are attainable for all addicts (except when it's a physical addiction and you need medical assistance). I absolutely believe that every addict, whether suffering from an addiction to pornograpy or overeating, social media or gaming, can stop his or her addiction for at least 24 hours. If you do it right, I am quite certain that you'll be able to add another 24 hours.

And another.

> **"When you make a conscious decision to quit your addiction, don't make it solely about the quitting itself; try to see what you could gain."**

Don't make it harder for yourself than it needs to be. Only the act of reaching that first milestone of 24 hours should give you a reason to celebrate. So celebrate if you've made it to the first 24 hours, celebrate again when you make it to 48 hours, and so on. Do this for at least one week. Find a healthy pleasure that isn't your addiction, like watching a movie with friends, taking a walk in nature, or buying yourself a little present. We'll discuss these options further in step 2.

I know the horrors of addiction. That's why the quitting process should be something wonderful. Of course there are lots of responsibilities to attend to after you've quit, like financial consequences, health problems, needing another diet, and deteriorated relationships. And of course, we'll deal with these problems in step 3. But there's more. When you make a conscious decision to quit your addiction, don't make it solely about the quitting itself; try to see what you could gain. A life of freedom, however you define that for yourself. Wearing that beautiful dress with confidence, being able to buy you friends dinner, being in a great condition, having a wonderful night out without being mean, because you're drunk or on drugs, and so on. That joyous and compelling dream or, when you haven't really defined your ideal life yet, at least the absence of addictive horrors will move you forward in the first days of quitting your addiction.

Seek help.

"Ask for help. Not because you are weak.
But because you want to remain strong."
Les Brown

When you've made the decision to quit, don't be alone. You could share your decision with the friend, family, professional worker or group you've contacted to talk about your addiction. Asking for help doesn't make you weak; it is the only smart way to know your weaknesses and give yourself the extra power of another person or support group to fight something as big as an addiction.

Define for yourself how you want to be helped. For example, the option of calling someone when you're having a really hard time with your addictive thoughts, having an accountability buddy, or simply ask the other person/support group what they suggest. For most addicts, it is one bridge too far to really seek professional help, and yes, there are other ways to do it. But it's going to be hard to do it all on your own. So at least share your story and find the courage to ask for help in whatever way suits you best. Like we went over in *Share your story*, you could also do it anonymously, online, or with a professional helpline.

Cut off resources.

What's critical in the quitting process is cutting off from resources that fuel your addiction. These could mean access to your money, to certain websites, to unhealthy food, alcohol, casinos, etc. By cutting yourself off from these resources, you will make it so much easier on yourself to actually follow through on your recovery. You could do this together with the person or group you've gone to for help.

When I made my final attempt to quit my gambling addiction, more than four years ago, I asked my good friend to take control of my bank account. He took over my banking passes and access to online banking. If you make it difficult for yourself to indulge in your addictive behaviour again, you have a better chance of succeeding.

If you want to you can find a healthy substitute for these resources. I still had some money, but it was cash money that my friend gave me. Or instead of bottles of wine, have bottles of a healthy soda you absolutely like, and so on. Don't change a bad habit for another bad habit. But use your imagination and pick something from the thousands of positive, healthy options this universe has to offer.

A Last word of Encouragement + Empowering Exercise

It's very easy to start blaming yourself during this period. It can be devastating thinking about all the problems you've caused with your addiction... Stop for a moment and consider your achievement of this day.

The day you quit. The day you stood up to your addiction. The day you said no the destructive and the decline and yes to a richer, more authentic life. To a new beginning.

You need to be your own best friend in this period (and for the rest of your life). Pat yourself on the back for taking this enormous step to committing to quitting your addiction forever. It's probably the most courageous thing you've done in your life so far.

Statements Exercise

A good way to emphasize this is by putting empowering statements/affirmations on sticky notes around your home or on your smartphone. There are countless free affirmation apps for your smartphone that can help you with this! A good exercise for now is to come up with at least 5 to 10 empowering statements/affirmations that will guide you through the initial stages of your recovery.

So why not do it right now. Sit down and write statements that speak to you.

Hereby a couple of examples:
There is so much more to life than the pain and suffering from addiction.

Addiction is a waste of my time.

Life in recovery is absolutely authentic for me.

Addiction is a lie, my spirit is the truth of recovery.

Addiction is killing my energy for life, recovery is my new energy.

The Universe/God is guiding me from the darkness of addiction into the light of recovery.

Recovery from the lies of addiction is my new way of life.

I am so much more than the destruction of addiction.

There are thousands of positive, creative options to spend your time on in life.

Only a fool waits for addiction to make him/her happy.

There are a lot of rules for affirmations, but just write down what **you feel is right**. Sometimes negative affirmations, such as 'Affirmation is killing my time', can be extremely helpful in the beginning stages of fighting an addiction. Especially when you mix it with positive statements.

The next level is to record your statements on your smartphone and listen to your statements/affirmations over and over again. When you go to work, when you cook, before you go to sleep, when you sleep, and so on. Change your thoughts, and you diminish the power of addiction significantly. To make it even better, you can put on some music under your statements. Search for 'audio mix' in the google play store or apple store to easily mix your statements with motivational music (instrumental music is highly recommended.

I added this exercise because, after the initial setup, it can be easily done without much effort. Just simply put in your earphones and go for a walk. Give your mind a different tape to listen to, than the destructive thought patterns of addiction. Listening to the statements can also bring up emotions, especially when you mix it with inspirational music (such as movie soundtracks). This can open up the possibility to release and confront the emotions around addiction. And find new passion, more intention for change.

Of course this statement exercise alone won't override your addictive thoughts. It's only a tool to help you during recovery. To emphasize where you don't want to go and where you *do* want to go. But you need more than affirmations to change. So we're going to find the patterns. To educate ourselves. To take responsibility. To find a new vision. And eventually we then can discover lasting change. So try out this exercise a couple of times for yourself, see how it works for you.

When it comes to recovery in general, there are no guru's. There are just teachers that can bring you to the truth within. Who can show you ways or methods to release thoughts, powers, that are holding back who you really are. The utmost reason why I would like you to try out this exercise is my belief that changing your thoughts almost always changes your reality. And, as all the exercises in this book have benefited me, this one especially has helped me enormously in my own recovery.

Summary – Step 1

- *Quitting your addiction? Do it smart.* Read the disclaimer of this book and the note to the reader.
- *Share your story.* Don't pull the full weight of your addiction all on your own. Find someone to share your story with.

- *Stop.* However you want to deal with your addiction, quitting it altogether first is the best way to conquer it. Stop and celebrate every day, for one week at least, that you've made this first step. Make it not only about quitting your addiction, but also about what you will gain when you quit.
- *Seek help.* In whatever way suits you best. It's really hard to quit totally on your own. *"Ask for help. Not because you are weak. But because you want to remain strong."*
- *Cutting off resources.* If you make it difficult for yourself to indulge in your addictive behaviour again, you have a better chance of succeeding.
- *Statements/affirmation exercise.* For changing your thoughts, almost always changes your reality.

End of this preview.

If you're interested in purchasing this workbook, you can go to amazon.com and find it there.

INSPIRATION

Books

Overcoming and understanding Addiction
Recovery: Freedom from Our Addictions by Russel Brand
Healing the Addicted Brain: The Revolutionary, Science-Based Alcoholism and Addiction Recovery Program by Harold Urschel
The Biology of Desire: why addiction is not a disease by Marc Lewis
The Disease to Please by Harriet B. Braiker
No More Mr. Nice Guy by Robert A. Glover
Born to Lose: Memoirs of a Compulsive Gambler by Bill Lee
The Power of Habit by Charles Duhigg
Quit Drinking by Joanne Edmund

Self growth (General)
Levels of Energy by Frederick Dodson
The Big Leap by Gay Hendricks
The Six Pillars of Self-Esteem by Nathaniel Branden
The Subtle Art of I Don't Give A Fuck by Mark Manson
The Slide Edge by Jeff Olson
Think and Grow Rich by Napoleon Hills
Outwitting the Devil by Napoleon Hills
Unleash the Power Within by Anthony Robbins
Feel The Fear And Do It Anyway by Susan Jeffers
The 4-Hour Workweek by Tim Ferris
The Underdog Advantage by Dean Graziosi
The 5 Second rule by Mel Robbins
The 7 Habits of Highly Successful People by Stephen R. Covey
No Excuses! The Power of Self-Discipline by Brian Tracey
The 12 Week Year by Brian P. Morgan
The War of Art, by Steven Pressfield
The 365 Self-Discovery Journal by 21 Exercises
The 5-Minute Gratitude Journal by Intelligent Change

Inspiring and Spiritual

The Power of Now by Eckhart Tolle
Energy Speaks: Messages from Spirit on Living, Loving, and Awakening by Lee Harris
The Little Prince by Antoine de Saint-Exupéry
The Prophet by Kahlil Gibran
The Portrait of Dorian Gray by Oscar Wilde
The Way of the Peaceful Warrior by Dan Millman
The Alchemist by Paulo Coelho
The Book Of Mastery by Paul Selig
Man's Search For Meaning by Victor Frankl
Ego is the Enemy by Ryan Holliday
100 Days Of Awakening, A Spiritual Journal by 21 Exercises
The Holy Man by Susan Trott

Finance

The Richest Man in Babylon by George Samuel Clason
Secrets of the Millionaire Mind by Harv Eker
Unshakeable: Your Financial Freedom Playbook by Anthony Robbins
Money Master The Game by Anthony Robbins
The Cashflow Quadrant by Robert Kiyosaki
Rich Dad Poor Dad by Robert Kiyosaki

Youtube

https://www.youtube.com/watch?v=dOkNkcZ_THA 5 Lessons To Live By - Dr. Wayne Dyer
https://www.youtube.com/user/LeeHarrisEnergy YouTube Channel Lee Harris, check out the 'Monthly Energy Updates'
https://www.youtube.com/watch?v=esdFGd5HcXQ Letting Go of Alcohol, Cigarettes and Drugs - Frederick Dodson
https://www.youtube.com/watch?v=RnFBz5QL9U0 Do This Every Morning For 17 Seconds Powerful Manifestation Tool - Abraham Hicks
https://www.youtube.com/watch?v=DLki68uLfjw Who We Are When We Are Not Addicted: The Possible Human - Dr. Gabor Maté
https://www.youtube.com/watch?v=zB8L9ZVFZj4 Having a Relapse? (Relapse Prevention, Recovery and How to Overcome Addiction Relapse) - Teal Swan

https://www.youtube.com/watch?v=dizQH0lxH6k Ohm Meditation
https://www.youtube.com/watch?v=LMmuChXra_M Ohm meditation for Sleep
https://www.youtube.com/watch?v=XSpVYtR6BVM Inner Smile Meditation for Self Love and Peace
https://www.youtube.com/watch?v=tw7XBKhZJh4 Waking Up with Sam Harris – Mindfulness Meditation (9 minutes)
https://www.youtube.com/watch?v=5MXpQYaekAA Raise Positive Vibration | 432Hz Healing Meditation | Energy Cleanse | Self Healing Frequency
https://www.youtube.com/watch?v=F28cryhKuQQ 963 hz / HIGHER SELF frequency / higher consciousness meditation, ask the universe for guidance

About The Author

C.W.V. Straaten is the author of *The Addiction Recovery Workbook, The Addiction Recovery Journal, Win The Morning Win The Day, The Gambling Addiction Recovery Journal* and *The Gambling Addiction Workbook*. After living in several countries, the author is now traveling the world, working on his inspiring self-help guides and a children's book.

You can reach mr. Van Straaten by email at cw.vanstraaten@yahoo.com. He doesn't do consulting, but he does read all his mail.

If you want to focus on becoming free from addiction & commit to recovery every day, follow my instagram account. With a recovery inspiration every day.

Instagram: become_recovery
https://www.instagram.com/become_recovery/.

Or you can search on C.W. V. Straaten.

Made in United States
Orlando, FL
11 November 2024